+10 WALL PILATES WORKOUTS

Transform Your Fitness Routine with Innovative Wall Pilates Exercises Workouts to Improve Your Flexibility, Tone Your Muscles, and Relieve Stress

CONTENTS

1: Introduction

2: Wall Roll Down

3: Wall Bridge

4: Wall Squat

5: Wall Push-Up

6: Wall Plank

7: Wall Leg Lift

8: Wall Side Kick

9: Wall Scissor Kicks

10: Wall Climb

11: Wall Standing Roll-Down

INTRODUCTION

A. Purpose and Goals of the Book:

Welcome to "+10 Wall Pilates Workouts," a comprehensive guide designed to introduce you to the transformative world of wall Pilates. This book aims to provide you with a structured, accessible, and effective approach to incorporating Pilates into your daily routine using the support of a wall. Whether you are a seasoned practitioner or a complete beginner, the goal of this book is to help you improve your fitness, enhance your well-being, and discover the myriad benefits of wall Pilates workouts.

Importance of Pilates for Fitness and Well-being:

Pilates is a powerful exercise regimen that emphasizes core strength, flexibility, balance, and body awareness. It is known for its ability to improve posture, reduce stress, and promote overall physical and mental health. By focusing on controlled movements and mindful breathing, Pilates helps to strengthen the body from the inside out, making it an ideal practice for people of all ages and fitness levels. The importance of Pilates in today's fast-paced world cannot be overstated, as it provides a sanctuary for the mind and body, fostering a sense of harmony and vitality.

Benefits of Wall Pilates Workouts:

Wall Pilates workouts bring a unique twist to traditional Pilates exercises by incorporating the stability and support of a wall. This added element helps to deepen stretches, enhance balance, and provide resistance, making the exercises more effective. The wall acts as a guide to ensure proper alignment and form, reducing the risk of injury and maximizing the benefits of each movement. With wall Pilates, you can expect improved muscle tone, increased flexibility, better posture, and a stronger core. Additionally, these workouts can be easily adapted to suit individual needs and fitness levels, making them a versatile and valuable addition to any exercise routine.

B. How to Use This Book:

Structure of the Book:

"+10 Wall Pilates Workouts" is carefully structured to guide you through a progressive series of workouts that build upon each other. The book is divided into chapters, each focusing on different aspects of wall Pilates. Starting with foundational exercises to establish a strong base, the workouts gradually increase in complexity and intensity. Each chapter includes detailed instructions, illustrated step-by-step guides, and tips to ensure you perform the exercises correctly and safely. The book also features variations and modifications to accommodate different fitness levels and goals.

Tips for Beginners:

If you are new to Pilates, this book provides all the guidance you need to start your journey confidently. Begin with the introductory chapters to familiarize yourself with the basic principles and fundamental exercises. Take your time to master the basics before moving on to more advanced workouts. Remember to listen to your body, progress at your own pace, and maintain consistent practice. Pay close attention to the alignment cues and breathing instructions provided in each exercise description, as these are crucial for achieving optimal results and preventing injury.

Necessary Equipment and Space Setup:

One of the great advantages of wall Pilates is that it requires minimal equipment and space. All you need is a sturdy wall, a comfortable exercise mat, and a small area where you can move freely. Ensure that the wall you choose is clear of any obstructions and provides enough support for the exercises. Having a mat will provide cushioning for your joints and help maintain a non-slip surface. Optional equipment such as resistance bands or small weights can be incorporated to add variety and challenge to your workouts, but they are not necessary for the basic routines.

THE WALL ROLL DOWN

The Wall Roll Down is a fundamental exercise in the Wall Pilates repertoire, offering a unique combination of flexibility, strength, and spinal articulation. This chapter delves into the nuances of the Wall Roll Down, providing a detailed description, step-by-step instructions, common mistakes, and variations to suit different fitness levels and goals.

A. Description and Benefits:

I. Detailed Explanation of the Exercise:

The Wall Roll Down is a Pilates exercise designed to enhance spinal flexibility, strengthen the core, and improve posture. By using a wall as support, this exercise allows practitioners to focus on controlled movements, ensuring proper alignment and engagement of the muscles. The exercise involves rolling the spine downwards, one vertebra at a time, and then rolling back up to a standing position, promoting spinal articulation and flexibility.

II. Muscles Targeted:

The Wall Roll Down primarily targets the following muscles:

Abdominals: Engages the rectus abdominis, transverse abdominis, and obliques for core stability.

Spinal Erectors: Activates the muscles along the spine to support spinal articulation.

Hip Flexors: Works the iliopsoas and other hip flexor muscles to facilitate movement.

Hamstrings: Stretches and engages the hamstrings, enhancing flexibility.

Glutes: Provides stability and support during the movement.

B. Step-by-Step Instructions:

I. Starting Position:

1. Stand against the wall: Position your back against a wall with your feet hip-width apart and about a foot away from the wall.

2. Align your spine: Ensure your head, shoulders, and back are in

contact with the wall. Your arms should hang naturally by your sides.

3. Engage your core: Activate your abdominal muscles to support your spine.

II. Movement Execution:

1. Inhale: Prepare for the movement by taking a deep breath in.

2. Exhale and roll down: Begin by tucking your chin towards your chest. Slowly start to peel your spine off the wall, vertebra by vertebra. Allow your arms to hang down as you roll forward.

3. Reach the bottom position: Continue rolling down until your

hands reach as close to the floor as possible, or until you feel a comfortable stretch in your hamstrings.

4. Inhale at the bottom: Pause briefly and take a deep breath in.

5. Exhale and roll up: Engage your core and start to roll back up, reversing the movement. Stack each vertebra back onto the wall, starting from your lower back and finishing with your head.

III. Tips for Proper Form and Alignment:

Move slowly and deliberately: Focus on controlled movements to ensure proper spinal articulation.

Engage your core: Keep your abdominal muscles engaged

throughout the exercise to support your spine.

Keep your knees soft: Avoid locking your knees; keep them slightly bent to prevent strain.

Breathe deeply: Coordinate your breath with your movements to enhance relaxation and control.

C. Common Mistakes and How to Avoid Them:

1. Rushing the Movement: Rolling down and up too quickly can compromise spinal articulation. Slow down and focus on each vertebra.

2. Overarching the Back: Maintain a natural curve in your spine.

Avoid overarching or flattening your back against the wall.

3. Locking the Knees: Keep a slight bend in your knees to prevent strain on your lower back and to facilitate movement.

4. Shallow Breathing: Deep, coordinated breathing is essential. Practice inhaling deeply and exhaling fully to enhance the movement.

D. Modifications and Variations:

Modifications:

1. Limited Flexibility: If you have limited flexibility, place a small cushion or yoga block under your

hands to reduce the range of motion.

2. Lower Back Sensitivity: If you experience discomfort in your lower back, reduce the depth of the roll down or keep your hands on your thighs for support.

Variations:

1. Wall Roll Down with Arm Circles: Add an upper body element by incorporating arm circles at the bottom of the roll down. This variation increases shoulder mobility and coordination.

2. Single Leg Roll Down: Lift one leg slightly off the ground and perform the roll down. This

variation challenges balance and engages the core more intensely.

3. Wall Roll Down with Resistance Band: Hold a resistance band in your hands and perform the roll down while maintaining tension in the band. This adds resistance and increases the challenge for your upper body and core.

The Wall Roll Down is a versatile exercise that can be adapted to suit various fitness levels and goals. By mastering this fundamental movement, you'll build a strong foundation for more advanced Wall Pilates exercises, enhance your spinal health, and improve your overall body awareness and control.

WALL BRIDGE

A. Description and Benefits:

The Wall Bridge is a highly effective Pilates exercise that leverages the stability of a wall to enhance the engagement of your core, glutes, and hamstrings. This exercise not only strengthens these muscle groups but also improves spinal mobility, posture, and overall balance. By incorporating the wall into this classic bridge exercise, you gain additional support, allowing for more precise movements and greater control. This makes the Wall Bridge an excellent choice for beginners and advanced practitioners alike.

I. Detailed Explanation of the Exercise:

The Wall Bridge involves lying on your back with your feet pressed against a wall. By lifting your hips towards the ceiling while keeping your feet stationary, you create a bridge shape with your body. This movement engages your core muscles to stabilize your spine, your glutes to lift your hips, and your hamstrings to maintain the bridge position. The wall provides a stable surface for your feet, helping to focus on muscle engagement and form without worrying about balance.

II. Muscles Targeted:

Core muscles: Including the rectus abdominis, transverse abdominis, and obliques, which stabilize your spine and maintain balance.

Glutes: The gluteus maximus, medius, and minimus are primarily responsible for lifting and maintaining the bridge.

Hamstrings: These muscles at the back of your thighs work to maintain the position of your legs and stabilize your pelvis.

Lower back muscles: Including the erector spinae, which help in spinal extension and maintaining the bridge position.

B. Step-by-Step Instructions:

I. Starting Position:

1. Lie on your back on a mat with your knees bent and feet flat on the floor.

2. Scoot closer to the wall until your feet can comfortably rest against it with your knees at a 90-degree angle.

3. Place your arms by your sides with palms facing down, and ensure your back is flat against the mat.

II. Movement Execution:

1. Inhale deeply to prepare.

2. As you exhale, engage your core by pulling your belly button towards your spine.

3. Press your feet firmly against the wall and slowly lift your hips off the mat, creating a straight line from your shoulders to your knees.

4. Hold the bridge position for a few seconds, ensuring that your glutes and hamstrings are fully engaged.

5. Inhale as you slowly lower your hips back to the mat with control.

6. Repeat the movement for 10-15 repetitions, maintaining proper form throughout.

III. Tips for Proper Form and Alignment:

Ensure your feet remain flat against the wall throughout the exercise.

Avoid arching your lower back; keep your core engaged to maintain a neutral spine.

Focus on lifting your hips using your glutes and hamstrings, not your lower back.

Keep your shoulders relaxed and your arms steady on the mat for support.

C. Common Mistakes and How to Avoid Them

1. Arching the Lower Back: This often happens if the core is not properly engaged. To avoid this, focus on pulling your belly button towards your spine and maintaining a neutral spine throughout the exercise.

2. Lifting Too High: Overextending your hips can place unnecessary strain on your lower back. Lift only to the point where

your body forms a straight line from shoulders to knees.

3. Feet Slipping on the Wall: Ensure that your feet are flat against the wall and not too high or too low. Adjust your position as needed to maintain stability.

4. Using the Lower Back Instead of the Glutes: Concentrate on squeezing your glutes and hamstrings to lift your hips, rather than pushing with your lower back.

D. Modifications and Variations:

Modifications:

1. For Beginners: If lifting your hips fully is too challenging, start

with smaller lifts. Gradually increase your range of motion as your strength improves.

2. Supported Bridge: Place a small cushion or rolled-up towel under your lower back for added support. This can help in maintaining a neutral spine and reducing strain.

Variations

1. Single-Leg Wall Bridge: Extend one leg straight out while performing the bridge with the other leg pressed against the wall. This increases the challenge and further engages the core and glutes.

2. Bridge with Heel Raises: Once in the bridge position, alternate

raising your heels off the wall. This variation adds an extra challenge to your calf muscles and balance.

3. Dynamic Wall Bridge: Instead of holding the bridge position, perform a series of controlled hip lifts and lowers. This adds a cardiovascular component and further strengthens the glutes and hamstrings.

Incorporating the Wall Bridge into your Pilates routine can provide a unique and effective way to strengthen your core, glutes, and hamstrings while improving overall stability and posture. With careful attention to form and alignment, this exercise can be adapted to suit various fitness levels and goals.

WALL SQUAT

A. Description and Benefits:

The wall squat is a fundamental exercise in Wall Pilates that combines the stability of a wall with the strength-building properties of a squat. This exercise is excellent for enhancing lower body strength, improving posture, and increasing overall stability. Wall squats can be modified to suit various fitness levels, making them an inclusive choice for anyone looking to build muscle and improve their fitness.

I. Detailed Explanation of the Exercise:

The wall squat involves leaning your back against a wall and lowering your body into a squat position, where your thighs are parallel to the ground. Unlike traditional squats, the wall provides support, which helps maintain proper form and alignment. This support allows you to focus on engaging your muscles effectively without the risk of tipping over or losing balance.

II. Muscles Targeted:

The wall squat primarily targets the quadriceps, hamstrings, glutes, and calves. Additionally, it engages the core muscles, including the rectus abdominis and obliques, to maintain stability and balance throughout the exercise.

B. Step-by-Step Instructions:

I. Starting Position:

1. Find a Clear Wall Space: Ensure there is enough space to perform the squat without any obstructions.

2. Stand Against the Wall: Position yourself with your back flat against the wall, feet hip-width apart and about two feet away from the wall.

3. Adjust Your Position: Slide down the wall slightly until your knees are bent at a comfortable angle, ensuring your knees are aligned with your ankles.

II. Movement Execution:

1. Begin the Squat: Slowly slide your back down the wall by bending your knees and lowering your body.

2. Achieve the Squat Position: Continue lowering until your thighs are parallel to the ground. Your knees should form a 90-degree angle, and your shins should be vertical.

3. Hold the Position: Maintain this position for the desired duration, typically starting with 15-30 seconds and gradually increasing as your strength improves.

4. Return to Starting Position: Push through your heels and straighten your legs to slide back up the wall to the starting position.

III. Tips for Proper Form and Alignment:

1. Maintain a Flat Back: Keep your back pressed against the wall throughout the exercise to ensure proper alignment.

2. Engage Your Core: Tighten your abdominal muscles to provide additional support and stability.

3. Knees Over Ankles: Ensure your knees stay directly above your ankles and do not extend past your toes.

4. Breathe Consistently: Inhale as you lower into the squat and exhale as you hold the position and return to standing.

C. Modifications and Variations:

I. Modifications for Beginners:

1. Partial Wall Squat: If a full squat is too challenging, start with a partial squat by lowering your body only halfway down the wall.

2. Shorter Hold Time: Begin with shorter hold times, such as 10-15 seconds, and gradually increase as you build strength and endurance.

3. Support with a Chair: Place a chair in front of you for additional support. Lightly hold the chair to help with balance while performing the wall squat.

II. Variations for Advanced Practitioners:

1. Single-Leg Wall Squat: Increase the difficulty by performing the

wall squat on one leg. Extend the other leg straight out in front of you while squatting and switch legs for the next set.

2. Wall Squat with Ball: Place an exercise ball between your back and the wall. This adds an element of instability, requiring more core engagement and balance.

3. Weighted Wall Squat: Hold dumbbells or a weighted plate while performing the wall squat to increase resistance and further challenge your muscles.

WALL PUSH-UP

A. Description and Benefits:

I. Detailed Explanation of the Exercise:

The wall push-up is a fundamental bodyweight exercise that leverages a wall for support. Unlike traditional floor push-ups, this variation reduces the load on your upper body, making it an excellent choice for beginners or those recovering from injuries. It provides a controlled environment to build strength, stability, and proper form before progressing to more challenging push-up variations.

II. Muscles Targeted:

The wall push-up primarily engages the following muscle groups:

Pectoralis Major: The main chest muscle responsible for the adduction and rotation of the upper arm.

Deltoids: The shoulder muscles, particularly the anterior (front) deltoids, which assist in arm flexion.

Triceps Brachii: The muscle on the back of the upper arm responsible for elbow extension.

Serratus Anterior: Located on the side of the chest, these muscles help with the upward rotation of the shoulder blade.

Core Muscles: Including the rectus abdominis and obliques,

which stabilize the torso during the exercise.

B. Step-by-Step Instructions

I. Starting Position:

1. Stand facing a wall with your feet hip-width apart.

2. Place your hands on the wall at shoulder height and shoulder-width apart. Your fingers should be pointing upward.

3. Walk your feet back slightly, ensuring that your body forms a straight line from head to heels. Your arms should be straight but not locked at the elbows.

II. Movement Execution:

1. Inhale: Begin by bending your elbows, keeping them close to your body, as you slowly lean toward the wall.

2. Lower your chest: Move your chest toward the wall until your elbows form a 90-degree angle.

3. Exhale: Push through your palms, straightening your arms to return to the starting position.

III. Tips for Proper Form and Alignment:

Maintain a straight line: Keep your body in a straight line from head to heels throughout the exercise. Avoid sagging your hips or arching your back.

Control your movement: Perform the push-up slowly and with control to maximize muscle engagement and reduce the risk of injury.

Engage your core: Tighten your abdominal muscles to help stabilize your body and support your spine.

C. Common Mistakes and How to Avoid Them:

1. Incorrect hand placement: Placing your hands too high or too wide can strain your shoulders. Ensure your hands are at shoulder height and shoulder-width apart.

2. Sagging hips: Letting your hips drop can lead to lower back strain.

Keep your core engaged to maintain a straight body line.

3. Locked elbows: Locking your elbows at the top of the movement can cause joint stress. Keep a slight bend in your elbows to maintain muscle tension.

D. Modifications and Variations:

1. Modified Wall Push-Up: For an easier variation, stand closer to the wall. This reduces the amount of body weight you need to push.

2. Single-Leg Wall Push-Up: To increase the challenge, lift one leg off the ground while performing the push-up. This adds an element of instability, engaging your core more intensely.

3. Incline Wall Push-Up: Place your hands higher up on the wall to decrease the angle between your body and the wall, making the exercise more challenging.

4. One-Arm Wall Push-Up: Perform the push-up with one arm to focus on unilateral strength and stability. Keep the other arm behind your back or at your side for balance.

WALL LEG LIFT

A. Description and Benefits:

I. Detailed Explanation of the Exercise:

The Wall Leg Lift is a fundamental exercise in Wall Pilates that focuses on enhancing lower body strength, stability, and flexibility. This exercise involves lifting one leg while maintaining support and alignment using a wall. It is an excellent move for engaging the core, improving balance, and sculpting the legs. By using the wall as a stabilizing force, practitioners can ensure proper form and alignment, making this exercise suitable for various fitness levels.

II. Muscles Targeted:

The Wall Leg Lift primarily targets the following muscle groups:

Quadriceps: Located at the front of the thigh, these muscles are responsible for knee extension.

Hamstrings: Situated at the back of the thigh, these muscles work to flex the knee and extend the hip.

Gluteus Maximus: This large muscle in the buttocks is essential for hip extension, outward rotation, and stabilization.

Hip Flexors: Including the iliopsoas, these muscles help lift the leg towards the torso.

Core Muscles: The abdominals and obliques are engaged to

maintain balance and stability during the movement.

B. Step-by-Step Instructions:

I. Starting Position:

1. Stand with your back against a wall, ensuring your heels are a few inches away from the wall.

2. Place your hands on your hips or extend them out to the sides for better balance.

3. Engage your core by drawing your navel towards your spine and ensure your shoulders are relaxed and down.

II. Movement Execution

1. Lift: Slowly lift one leg straight up in front of you, aiming to bring it to hip height or higher if flexibility allows. Keep the leg extended and toes pointed.

2. Hold: Pause briefly at the top of the movement, maintaining balance and ensuring the lifted leg is straight and the supporting leg is stable.

3. Lower: Gradually lower the leg back down to the starting position with control, avoiding any sudden movements.

4. Repeat: Perform the desired number of repetitions on one leg before switching to the other leg.

III. Tips for Proper Form and Alignment:

Keep your back pressed firmly against the wall to avoid arching.

Maintain a slight bend in the supporting leg to protect the knee joint.

Ensure the lifted leg remains straight without locking the knee.

Engage the core throughout the exercise to maintain balance and stability.

Breathe steadily, exhaling during the lift and inhaling during the lowering phase.

C. Common Mistakes and How to Avoid Them:

1. Arching the Back: Ensure your back remains flat against the wall. Engage your core muscles to support proper spinal alignment.

2. Locking the Knee: Avoid locking the knee of the lifted leg. Maintain a slight bend to prevent strain on the joint.

3. Rushing the Movement: Perform the exercise slowly and with control to maximize muscle engagement and reduce the risk of injury.

4. Improper Foot Position: Point your toes and keep the foot of the lifted leg in a neutral position to ensure correct muscle activation.

D. Modifications and Variations:

1. Modification for Beginners:

If lifting the leg to hip height is challenging, start with a lower lift, gradually increasing the height as strength and flexibility improve.

Use a chair or wall for additional balance support if needed.

2. Variation for Advanced Practitioners:

Wall Leg Lift with Ankle Weights: Add ankle weights to increase resistance and intensify the workout.

Wall Leg Lift with Pulses: At the top of the lift, perform small pulsing movements to further engage the muscles and increase the challenge.

Single-Leg Wall Squat with Leg Lift: Combine a single-leg wall squat with the leg lift for a compound movement that targets multiple muscle groups.

WALL SIDE KICK

A. Description and Benefits:

The Wall Side Kick is a Pilates exercise that emphasizes stability, strength, and flexibility. By using the wall as support, this exercise ensures proper alignment and enhances the engagement of the core, glutes, and legs. This move not only strengthens the lower body but also improves balance and coordination.

I. Detailed Explanation of the Exercise:

The Wall Side Kick is performed by positioning yourself sideways to a wall, using the wall for support and balance. The exercise involves lifting and extending one leg to the side while maintaining a stable and aligned core. This movement challenges the muscles to maintain stability and control, promoting strength and flexibility.

II. Muscles Targeted:

Gluteus Medius and Minimus: These muscles are primarily responsible for hip abduction and stabilization during the side kick.

Hip Flexors: Engaged to lift the leg.

Quadriceps and Hamstrings: Support the leg movement and stability.

Core Muscles: Including the obliques, to maintain balance and alignment.

Adductors: Assist in controlling the leg movement back to the starting position.

B. Step-by-Step Instructions:

I. Starting Position:

1. Stand sideways to a wall with your feet hip-width apart.

2. Place the hand closest to the wall on it for support at shoulder height.

3. Ensure your body is straight, with shoulders and hips aligned.

4. Engage your core, pulling your navel towards your spine.

II. Movement Execution:

1. Lift and Extend:

Inhale deeply.

As you exhale, lift your outer leg (the one furthest from the wall) to the side, keeping it straight.

Extend your leg out as high as you can while maintaining balance and alignment.

Hold your leg at the top for a brief moment.

2. Return to Start:

Inhale as you slowly lower your leg back to the starting position.

Maintain control and stability throughout the movement.

3. Repetitions:

Perform 10-15 repetitions on one side before switching to the other.

III. Tips for Proper Form and Alignment

Maintain a Neutral Spine: Avoid arching your back or leaning forward. Keep your spine neutral and straight.

Engage the Core: Continuously engage your core muscles to support your lower back and maintain balance.

Controlled Movements: Focus on slow and controlled movements to maximize muscle engagement and avoid injury.

Breathing: Coordinate your breathing with your movements; inhale during preparation and exhale during the kick.

C. Common Mistakes and How to Avoid Them:

1. Leaning Forward or Backward:

Mistake: Leaning forward or backward instead of maintaining a straight posture.

Solution: Engage your core and focus on keeping your shoulders and hips aligned.

2. Dropping the Leg Too Quickly:

Mistake: Allowing the leg to drop quickly rather than controlling the descent.

Solution: Concentrate on a slow, controlled return to the starting position.

3. Arching the Back:

Mistake: Arching the back excessively during the leg lift.

Solution: Keep the spine neutral and avoid overarching by engaging the core.

4. Insufficient Core Engagement:

Mistake: Not engaging the core muscles sufficiently, leading to instability.

Solution: Focus on drawing the navel towards the spine and maintaining core tension throughout the exercise.

D. Modifications and Variations:

Modifications:

1. Reduced Range of Motion:

If you find it challenging to lift your leg high, reduce the range of motion. Lift your leg only as high as you can while maintaining proper form.

2. Additional Support:

Place a chair beside you for extra support if needed. This can help you maintain balance and build strength gradually.

Variations:

1. Wall Side Kick with Resistance Band:

Add a resistance band around your ankles to increase the intensity. This variation targets the muscles more deeply and enhances strength.

2. Wall Side Kick Pulse:

Instead of a single lift, perform small pulsing movements at the top of the kick. This variation increases muscle endurance and adds a challenge.

3. Wall Side Kick with Arm Extension:

Extend the arm opposite to the kicking leg straight out to the side. This variation enhances balance and engages the upper body muscles.

Incorporating the Wall Side Kick into your Pilates routine offers numerous benefits, from strengthening key muscles to improving balance and coordination. By following the detailed instructions and focusing on proper form, you can maximize the effectiveness of this exercise and avoid common mistakes. Don't hesitate to modify or vary the exercise to suit your fitness level and goals.

WALL SCISSOR KICKS

A. Description and Benefits:

Wall Scissor Kicks are a dynamic and challenging exercise that utilizes the wall for support and stability. This exercise not only engages multiple muscle groups but also enhances coordination and flexibility. Incorporating Wall Scissor Kicks into your Pilates routine can help improve core strength, leg power, and overall body alignment.

I. Detailed Explanation of the Exercise:

Wall Scissor Kicks involve alternating leg movements while maintaining a stable core and a firm connection with the wall. The exercise mimics a scissor-like motion with the legs, targeting both the lower and upper body. It requires precise control and balance, making it an excellent addition to any Pilates workout for enhancing functional fitness.

II. Muscles Targeted:

Wall Scissor Kicks primarily target the following muscle groups:

Core Muscles: Including the rectus abdominis, transverse abdominis, and obliques.

Hip Flexors: Particularly the iliopsoas.

Quadriceps: Front of the thighs.

Hamstrings: Back of the thighs.

Adductors and Abductors: Inner and outer thigh muscles.

Gluteus Maximus: Buttocks muscles.

B. Step-by-Step Instructions:

I. Starting Position

1. Stand with your back against the wall, ensuring your entire spine is in contact with the surface.

2. Place your hands on your hips or extend them out to the sides for additional balance.

3. Walk your feet forward until your body forms a slight angle with the wall, maintaining contact

with your upper back and shoulders.

II. Movement Execution:

1. Engage your core by drawing your navel towards your spine.

2. Lift your right leg straight up in front of you, keeping it as straight as possible.

3. Simultaneously, lower your left leg straight down, keeping it just above the floor without touching it.

4. Switch legs by lifting your left leg up and lowering your right leg down, performing a controlled scissor motion.

5. Continue alternating legs for the desired number of repetitions,

maintaining a steady pace and ensuring smooth transitions.

III. Tips for Proper Form and Alignment:

Keep Your Core Engaged: Maintain core activation throughout the exercise to stabilize your spine and prevent lower back strain.

Maintain a Neutral Spine: Ensure your lower back does not arch away from the wall.

Control Your Movements: Avoid swinging your legs. Instead, focus on slow, deliberate motions.

Breathe Consistently: Inhale as you prepare, exhale as you perform the movement, and maintain a steady breathing rhythm.

Avoid Locking Your Knees: Keep a slight bend in your knees to prevent joint strain.

C. Common Mistakes and How to Avoid Them:

1. Arching the Lower Back: To avoid this, engage your core and ensure your lower back remains in contact with the wall.

2. Swinging the Legs: Focus on controlled, deliberate movements rather than relying on momentum.

3. Improper Foot Position: Keep your feet flexed or pointed consistently, avoiding any random foot positioning.

4. Tension in the Neck and Shoulders: Relax your upper body and focus on the movement of your legs.

D. Modifications and Variations:

Modifications:

1. Reduced Range of Motion: If you're a beginner or have limited flexibility, perform the exercise with a smaller range of motion, gradually increasing as you become more comfortable.

2. Bent Knee Version: Perform the exercise with slightly bent knees to reduce the intensity and strain on the hamstrings and lower back.

Variations:

1. Single-Leg Wall Scissor Kicks: Perform the exercise with one leg at a time, focusing on slow and controlled movements to enhance strength and stability.

2. Resistance Band Scissor Kicks: Place a resistance band around your thighs or ankles to add extra resistance and intensity to the exercise.

3. Elevated Scissor Kicks: Perform the exercise with your upper back elevated on a stability ball to increase the challenge to your core and balance.

WALL CLIMB

A. Description and Benefits:

I. Detailed Explanation of the Exercise:

The Wall Climb is a dynamic Pilates exercise that leverages the support and resistance of a wall to enhance strength, stability, and flexibility. This exercise involves using your body's weight and the wall's resistance to create a full-body workout. It mimics the motion of climbing but with the added benefit of wall support, making it accessible and challenging for individuals of various fitness levels.

II. Muscles Targeted:

The Wall Climb primarily targets the following muscle groups:

Core: Engages the abdominal muscles, particularly the rectus abdominis and obliques, to maintain stability and control.

Upper Body: Works the shoulders, biceps, triceps, and upper back muscles to pull and push the body up and down the wall.

Lower Body: Activates the glutes, quadriceps, hamstrings, and calves to stabilize and support the body's movements.

B. Step-by-Step Instructions:

I. Starting Position:

1. Stand facing the wall with your feet hip-width apart.

2. Place your hands flat on the wall at shoulder height, fingers pointing upwards.

3. Step back slightly to allow your body to lean into the wall at an angle, creating a straight line from your head to your heels.

II. Movement Execution:

1. Climbing Up:

Engage your core and press firmly into the wall with your hands.

Slowly walk your hands up the wall, one hand at a time, while simultaneously walking your feet closer to the wall.

Continue this coordinated movement until your hands are as high as comfortable and your body forms a diagonal line with the wall.

2. Climbing Down:

Reverse the motion by walking your hands down the wall, one at a time.

Step your feet back to maintain the angle and control as you descend.

Continue until you return to the starting position.

III. Tips for Proper Form and Alignment:

Maintain Core Engagement: Keep your abdominal muscles engaged throughout the exercise to support your lower back and maintain stability.

Control Your Movement: Perform the exercise slowly and with

control to maximize muscle engagement and minimize the risk of injury.

Alignment: Ensure that your body forms a straight line from your head to your heels, avoiding arching or sagging at the hips.

Breathing: Inhale as you prepare and exhale as you climb up or down the wall, maintaining a steady breathing pattern.

C. Common Mistakes and How to Avoid Them:

1. Arching the Back: Allowing the lower back to arch can strain the lumbar spine.

Solution: Engage your core muscles and focus on keeping a

neutral spine throughout the exercise.

2. Rushing the Movement: Moving too quickly can compromise form and increase the risk of injury.

Solution: Perform the exercise slowly and deliberately, focusing on muscle engagement and control.

3. Incorrect Hand Placement: Placing hands too wide or too narrow can affect stability and effectiveness.

Solution: Keep your hands shoulder-width apart and ensure even pressure on the wall.

4. Lack of Core Engagement: Failing to engage the core can lead to poor posture and reduced effectiveness.

Solution: Consistently activate your core muscles to support your movements and maintain proper alignment.

D. Modifications and Variations:

Modifications:

1. Assisted Wall Climb: For beginners, start with your feet closer to the wall and your body more upright to reduce the intensity.

2. Partial Climb: Limit the range of motion by only climbing halfway

up the wall before returning to the starting position.

Variations:

1. Single-Leg Wall Climb: Perform the climb with one leg lifted, alternating legs to increase the challenge and engage the core and lower body more intensely.

2. Wall Climb with Resistance Band: Attach a resistance band to your wrists and perform the wall climb, adding resistance to the upper body and intensifying the workout.

3. Wall Climb with Leg Lifts: Incorporate leg lifts during the climb by lifting one leg off the ground as you climb up and down, alternating legs to further engage the lower body and core.

WALL STANDING ROLL-DOWN

A. Description and Benefits:

I. Detailed explanation of the exercise:

The Wall Standing Roll-Down is a foundational Pilates exercise designed to improve spinal articulation and flexibility while enhancing overall posture and core strength. It involves controlled movement through the spine, engaging deep core muscles for stability and support.

II. Muscles targeted:

Core muscles: Rectus abdominis, transverse abdominis, obliques.

Spinal muscles: Erector spinae, multifidus.

Shoulder and upper back muscles: Rhomboids, trapezius.

This exercise promotes lengthening and decompression of the spine, helping to alleviate tension and improve mobility in the upper back and shoulders.

B. Step-by-Step Instructions:

I. Starting position:

1. Stand with your back against a wall, feet hip-width apart, and a slight bend in your knees.

2. Engage your abdominal muscles by drawing your navel towards your spine.

3. Ensure your shoulders are relaxed away from your ears with your arms by your sides.

II. Movement execution:

1. Inhale to prepare.

2. Exhale as you slowly nod your chin towards your chest, initiating the movement from the top of your head.

3. Continue to articulate your spine downward, one vertebra at a time, as if peeling your spine off the wall.

4. Maintain contact with the wall as long as possible while rolling down towards the floor.

5. Pause briefly at the bottom of the movement with your hands hanging towards the floor and your head between your arms.

III. Tips for proper form and alignment:

Keep your knees soft throughout the movement to avoid locking them.

Maintain a neutral pelvis position; avoid tucking or tilting excessively.

Imagine lengthening your spine as you roll down, rather than collapsing forward.

Focus on breathing deeply and smoothly throughout the exercise to facilitate movement and relaxation.

C. Common Mistakes and How to Avoid Them:

Rounding the shoulders: Focus on keeping the shoulders relaxed and away from the ears.

Collapsing through the spine: Maintain core engagement to support each vertebra as you roll down.

Holding the breath: Remember to breathe continuously, especially during the descent.

D. Modifications and Variations

Modification: If standing against the wall is challenging, perform the exercise standing away from the wall, focusing on maintaining alignment.

Variation: Add a challenge by using a small Pilates ball between your knees to engage inner thigh muscles and enhance stability.

The Wall Standing Roll-Down is an effective exercise for improving posture, enhancing spinal flexibility, and building core strength. Practice it regularly to experience greater mobility and alignment in your daily activities.

www.ingramcontent.com/pod-product-compliance
Lightning Source LLC
Chambersburg PA
CBHW071841210526
45479CB00001B/230